Fast, Simple & Fresh Gluten Free
Recipes for Soups & Appetizers
Deliciously Engineered for Weight Loss

by Jaqui Karr, c.s.n., c.v.d.

check out Jaqui's fun online nutrition club at:

http://JaquiKarr.com/TheParty

Wish you could attend Jaqui's gluten seminar?
Go to: GlutenDemystified.com

GW00693974

As a nutrition expert, I know where people usually go wrong in their diet. **As a foodie,** *I understand.* **As a gluten expert,** I am on high alert for the poisons people are unknowingly putting into their bodies.

These recipes are designed to solve 3 problems at once and do it in a fantastically delicious way!

Since soups and appetizers are not the main meal it can be easy to forget their importance. The fact is that a nutritionally dense and really satisfying starter is going to automatically cause you to eat less and provide a ton of vitamins & minerals at the same time.

I won't talk about gluten sensitivity in any detail here since I have a book that does that and after all, this is just all about the food! But I will say that whether you are intolerant to gluten or not, eating food that supercharges your immune system is always a great thing!

We could ALL use boosts to our immune system – it is our body's #1 defense mechanism against pretty much every disease possible.

These particular dishes are all absolutely guaranteed to be 100% free of gluten, dairy, sugar, peanuts, shellfish, and soy because they are completely raw dishes. Not only does that make them the safest food to eat for anyone with food allergies, it also makes these dishes the most nutritionally dense possible.

The best part? Everything takes just minutes to make and so full of flavor that you'll forget they're so good for you!

All that's left to say is: *enjoy!*

Jaqui Karr

DELICIOUS SIMPLICITY

I often create dishes with rich flavors, sometimes very spicy, sometimes strong blends, which makes it nice to cleanse the palate between courses or even before starting the meal. What better place to start our recipes?

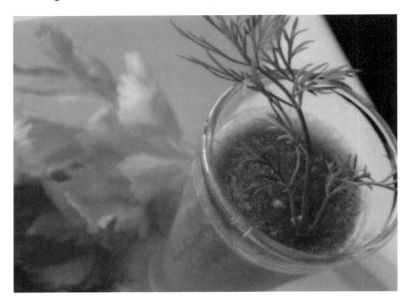

IN A BLENDER, equal amounts:

celery
cucumber
dill
water

Serve in a shot glass if you intend to serve it just once, or use a tiny bowl or even coffee cup to leave it on the table so you may take a sip from it as desired throughout the meal (include 2 ice cubes as it is nicer when chilled)

Leftover green mix? Soup – of course.

Though considering the anti-aging properties of this mixture, you might want to just make a soup or tall drink out of it in the first place.

When making it as a soup, replace the water with coconut water - this will add a variance of flavor and also add potassium & electrolytes & more. And sprinkle organic coconut flakes on top.

As always, make sure your ingredients are organic – but specifically the cucumber here because you definitely want to leave the peel on for all the wonderful anti-aging properties.

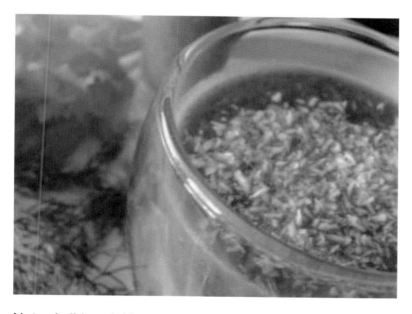

Note: I did sprinkle coconut flakes for this photo, which I would do when using the recipe as a soup, but not as a palate cleanser as it does add an element of sweetness.

BLACK BEAN SOUP

(even beans can be elegant!)

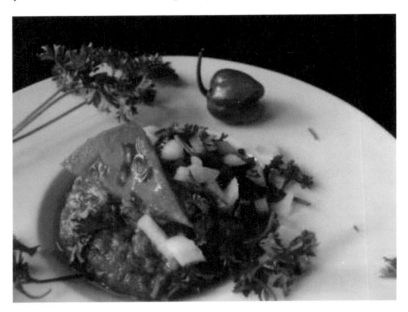

IN BLENDER:

1 cup black beans (soaked or cooked)
1 large tomato or 2 small such as plum
2 tbsp tomato paste
1 small white onion
1 cup parsley (can be blended in or chopped on top as shown here)
2 tsps cumin powder
1 tsp dried oregano or small bunch fresh oregano
1 small hot pepper (omit for mild version)
1/3 cup water

WHY YOU WANT TO EAT BLACK BEANS

1 cup of black beans: 15g fiber, 15g protein, 181mg omega-3's, 46mg calcium, 3.6mg iron, 1.9mg zinc, 0.4mg copper, 120mg magnesium, 0.8mg manganese, 241mg phosphorus, 611mg potassium, 256mcg folate, 0.4mg thiamin

...and this is just the list of nutrients in significant amounts, there are trace amounts of more, plus the nutrients scientists haven't discovered yet...

SOAKING BEANS

Not really necessary because cooked beans actually do manage to keep their nutritional content intact. You definitely want to avoid canned beans (or any food) when possible, so do try to buy dried beans and cook them yourself. If you absolutely can't avoid canned, find organic that specifies "BPA free" on the can – at a minimum you want to avoid that harmful toxin.

If you want to try soaking it is as easy as this:

In a glass container put beans and pure clean water, leave to soak overnight at room temperature. Pour into a strainer and soak thoroughly, put beans back into the glass container and soak again with fresh clean water.

Repeat this process morning and evening for 3-5 days (taste one after the 3rd day to see if you like it; I generally soak 5 days), and you're all set.

BROCCOLI STALK SOUP and then some!

We love using broccoli florets for dips and snacks, but what happens to the poor stalks? Get the blender out and let's make some soup! Of course you can use the entire broccoli - this is just to give you an idea of what to do with the portion of broccoli you may have been throwing out.

One of the most fabulous things about all green soups is how well other flavors blend with them. Instead of blending everything together (where you'll end up with a gazpacho), try making the soup with just the greens and chop everything else over it like I have here... this way you will get the true flavor of every wonderful fresh ingredient.

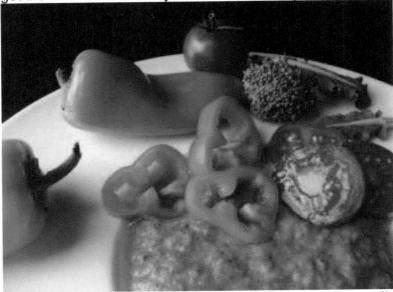

IN BLENDER OR FOOD PROCESSOR: 2 cups broccoli stalks, 1 cup parsley, 1 zucchini, 1-2 cloves garlic, 2 tbsp lemon juice, 1 cup water, black pepper and salt to taste **Note:** you do want to eat this immediately; it is not a great prep-ahead recipe because it is so high in water content that it will break down in texture pretty quickly

...WE HAVE OUR BASE BROCCOLI SOUP... *AND NOW WE PLAY...*

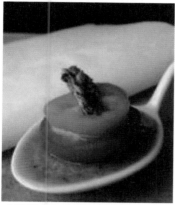

AMUSE BOUCHE - You can layer with anything to make a fun little amuse bouche. Using contrasting colors like red, orange, and yellow will make it extra fun (and add a whole other variety of nutrients). Here I have a spoon of the soup, tomato, sweet yellow pepper, topped with a tiny piece of flax & sunflower seed cracker for texture

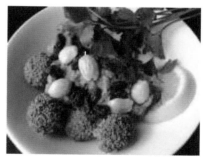

STARTER SAUCE - I was really craving broccoli here, so I used the soup as a sauce and poured over broccoli florets – you can pour over anything. I also added cayenne pepper to the soup and then to balance the heat I added sweet raisins, and finally for a crunchy texture I added truffled salted almonds. This simple variation came out fantastic! One simple recipe, 3 great variations.

CELERY & WATERCRESS SOUP

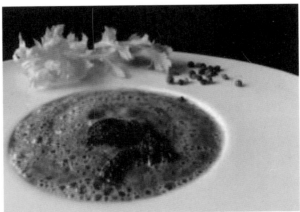

IN FOOD PROCESSOR or BLENDER:
1 cup chopped celery
1 cup chopped cucumber
2 cups tightly packed watercress
½ cup carrots
¼ cup sun dried tomatoes or raisins to top
1 cup water
1 tsp nutritional yeast (gluten free)
Salt and black pepper to taste
TIP: make it more fun by serving in a martini glass – beautifully elegant when entertaining!

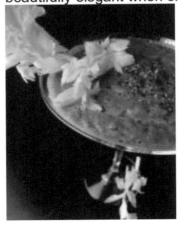

SUN DRIED TOMATO & WATERMELON

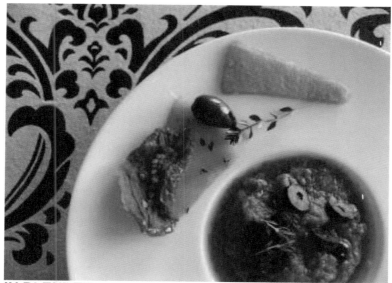

IN BLENDER:

3 cups cold watermelon (or add some ice cubes if it is at room temperature)

3/4 cup sun dried tomatoes

1 tsp cayenne pepper (or paprika)

1 tbsp thyme

Top with chopped black olives or hemp seeds or both!

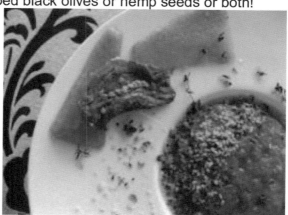

CARROT & AVOCADO SOUP

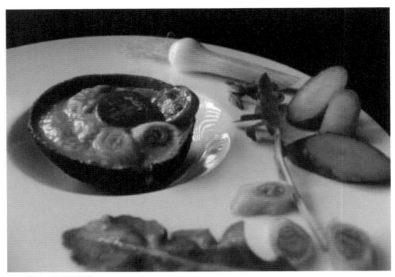

IN BLENDER:

3 carrots (any color)
1 avocado (can substitute with 1 zucchini)
1 cup coriander (spinach or arugula are great options too)
1 cup water
1 green onion
1 clove garlic
1 tbsp nutritional yeast
1 tsp cumin powder
½ tsp salt
Juice of 1 lime
Freshly cracked black pepper

NOTE: I have shown the recipe in a simple clean presentation, but to pile on the nutrients I suggest topping with large portions of chopped greens like spinach or parsley, red peppers, and any other vegetable or herb you might wish to add. Recipes like this are a perfect base that you can very easily add anything to!

ARUGULA SOUP

Incredibly simple ingredients, amazingly rich taste. I credit the peppery taste of the arugula.

IN BLENDER:

4 cups arugula
1 green tomato
3-4 sun dried tomatoes
3-4 sprigs of thyme
2 tbsp flax seed oil (any oil)
2 drops balsamic vinegar (adjust this amount according to how aged your balsamic vinegar is; the 20 year Modena I am using is extremely potent, the ones in most pantries probably require an adjustment from ½ to 1 tsp)
Optional: teaspoon ground flax or hemp
Add water to desired thickness, salt and pepper to taste

This takes just 2 minutes to make and you will have added a terrific serving of greens to your meal!

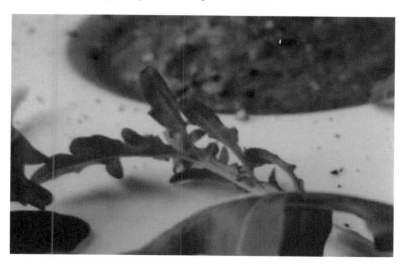

INSPIRATION

You never know where inspiration for a dish comes from. Sometimes it is the main ingredient itself and other times it is just something you want to chop into or on top of your dish. Today my favorite grower at the farmer's market had the most fantastic carrots and I knew I wanted to make a dish where their wondrous colors would not get lost.

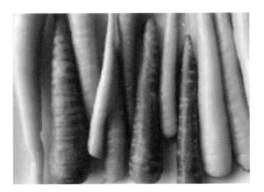

Mandolin or a knife, try cutting at different angles to create interesting shapes – it makes for fantastic presentation. …but don't wait until you are entertaining to do this! Do it for yourself as often as you can and add another layer of enjoyment to your meals! THIS PAGE: bits & pieces of our soup toppings served on basil leaf

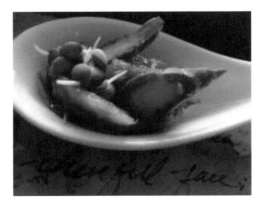

SPROUTED LENTIL & TOMATO SOUP

...as a starter, soup in a bowl, snack in a cup, or elegant appetizers

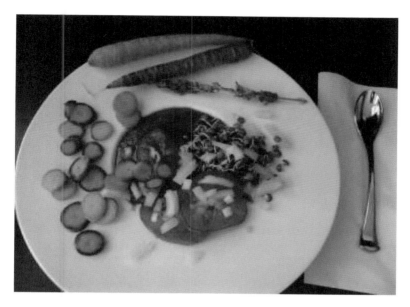

IN BLENDER:
3 cups raw or cooked tomatoes
2 tbsp tomato paste
½ tsp salt
1 tsp paprika
1 tsp oregano

So now you have your base, you are ready to create a unique masterpiece each time with whatever you want to chop into it. I love carrots, bell peppers, and even mushrooms. I must mention that beans and sprouts go exceptionally well with tomato soup and from a nutrition point of view add so much, so try to incorporate them into dishes often.

SPROUTING LENTILS

...this is one of those situations where you will find yourself saying "if I had known it was THAT easy, I would have been doing this years ago." *It IS that easy.*

Rinse 1 cup of brown lentils (any variety) then soak in pure clean cool water (60-70°) overnight (minimum 12 hours, you don't need to be exact). 3 cups water per cup of lentils.

Strain and rinse (always cool water) until the rinse water is completely clear. Many begin the sprouting at this stage, I like to soak a second time for another 12 hours, so just repeat above or skip to the next step which is to pour the lentils into a mason jar (any container will do) and cover the top with a cheese cloth or any cloth that allows for aeration. Then twice a day rinse the lentils and put back into your jar and again cover the top with a cheese cloth.

Repeat this process 2-3 days until you see little leaves sprouting out of each lentil. You can sprout up to 6 days if you wish, this will just create larger sprouts; to avoid over or under-sprouting I suggest 3-4 days. Once sprouted they are ready to eat; transfer to a container and store them in the refrigerator if not using them all immediately. They can keep for days and are a fantastic base as well as a terrific food to sprinkle over other dishes.

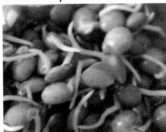

TURMERIC & LENTIL STARTER

TURMERIC: One of the most amazing foods on earth and we use it far too rarely! An amazing anti-inflammatory with a really long list of benefits. Studies are ongoing but shown to be the #1 defense against Alzheimer's disease.

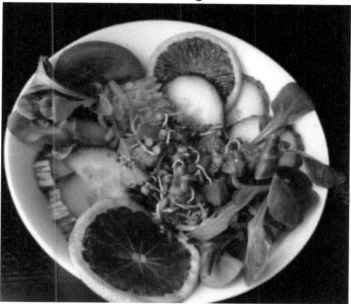

I like this particular base for very specific* reasons:
--Sliced English cucumber (*cooling, counters the spice)
--Shredded carrots (*to add sweetness)
--Mâché greens (*for their light flavor, spinach or any lettuce would work just as well)
TOPPING: 1 cup sprouted lentils 1 plum tomato diced (any tomato is fine), freshly squeezed juice of 1 blood orange and ¾ tsp turmeric. **TIP:** if you aren't used to the flavor of turmeric, it could take getting used to... a great tip is to always mix with sweet flavors like carrots, mango, oranges, raisins, or apples.

MANGO & TURMERIC

This is about as easy as it gets – just minutes to make – and the flavors were MADE to be together!

Chop up whatever greens you have, I am using kale & collards here, but I have done this with brussel sprouts, broccoli, asparagus, and every other green on earth. The mango stays the same, the greens always change.

Chop up some sweet champagne (yellow) mango (perfect balance to the spicy turmeric), sprinkle turmeric (also called curcumin) and add a few drops of water or to make it sweeter, the juice of an orange, to help dissolve & mix the turmeric in and you're set – the perfect fast starter.

This simple mix contains a potent dose of nutrients, antioxidants, anti-inflammatories, beta-carotene,…

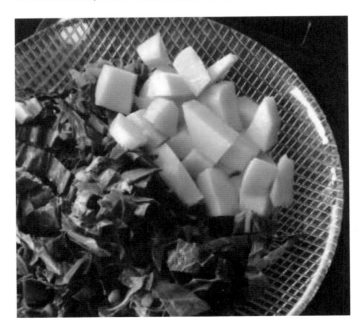

TOMATO CELEBRATION APPETIZERS

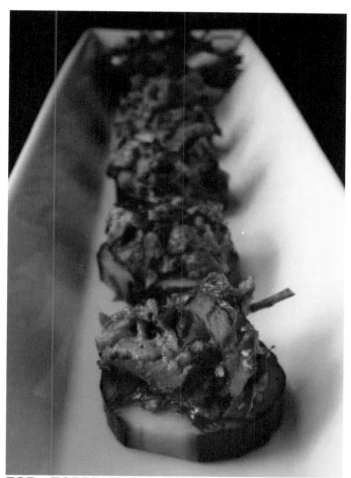

FOR TOPPING, IN FOOD PROCESSOR: 2 fresh tomatoes, 5oz sun dried tomatoes, 3oz green olives, 2 cloves garlic, juice of 1 lime, 3 tbsp ground flax, 1 tbsp nutritional yeast, 2 tsps olive oil; optional 1 cup parsley, purslane, or coriander (chopped and hand mixed in when serving as appetizer or in wrap). Serve on vegetables or your favorite crackers!

WHY YOU WANT TO EAT SPROUTS

Let's start with: sprouts retard the aging process (that's enough info for most people to want to eat them) but let's know more, I'm giving you the super condensed version:

--sprouts are a living bio-genic food which means they strongly support the regeneration of cells in your body

--they contain something most foods don't have: oxygen (two time Nobel Prize winner Dr. Otto Warbur said he found cancer cells to be initiated by lack of oxygen)

--they are an alkaline food and do a terrific job of raising our body's alkaline level

--they provide EFA's (essential fatty acids), fiber, chlorophyll (powerful blood cleanser), and a whole array of other vitamins and minerals (which vary from variety to variety of sprouts, so keep alternating)

An extremely nutritionally dense food with such few calories, low on the glycemic index, and incredibly easy to incorporate into meals every day! Throw them into green smoothies, salads, chop them up over soups, layer into raw lasagna, put them into sandwiches…

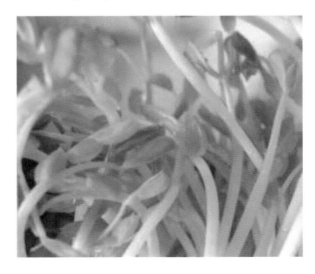

TOMATO SPROUT TOWER

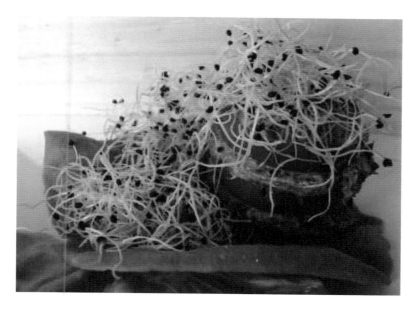

THE FILLING, IN A FOOD PROCESSOR:
2 cups kale
1 cup purslane (or spinach)
1 cup broccoli
juice of 1 lemon & rinds
1/2 cup walnuts
1/2 cup tahini
3 tbsp ground flaxseeds
1 tbsp cumin powder
1 tbsp nutritional yeast

NOTE: you definitely do not want to skip the ground flax seeds because that is what makes the mixture thick enough to hold your tower in place. You can even add more than the quantity I have placed in the recipe.

TOMATO: I love the big hothouse tomatoes for this, those vine ripened (as shown here) works fine

PEPPER BOAT APPETIZERS

We've talked about how fantastic sprouts are. We've talked about how fantastic black beans are. Now let's put them together!

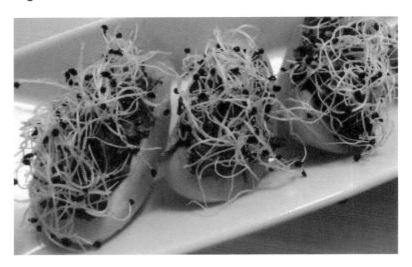

TOSS GENTLY:
2 cups black beans
2 cups chopped parsley (or cilantro)
1 large tomato diced
2 green onions chopped (any onion works)
2 cloves of mashed garlic
1 tbsp cayenne pepper
½ tsp black pepper
juice of 1 lime (any citrus*)
4 tbsp flaxseed oil
Optional: ½ cup shredded dulse (or any sea vegetable)

TIP: *you always want to add lemon, lime, or orange juice to the mix because vitamin C improves your body's ability to absorb the iron in the beans.

CHERRY TOMATO BOMBS

What makes these gorgeous little appetizers bombs?
The nutrient dense power in them!

IN THE FOOD PROCESSOR:
2 cups kale
2 cups dandelion (flowers too if you have them)
1 cup purslane
½ cup rapini
½ cup spinach
1 cup any sea vegetable, I like dulse
2 carrots
1 entire orange or juice of 1 lemon*
1 tbsp cayenne pepper
2 tbsp tahini
3 tbsp ground flax
--SPOON into little cherry tomatoes (carve out tomatoes with melon baller first and add to the mixture)

TIP: *When using a bitter green like dandelion, if you are not used to the flavor, add sweetness by using a whole orange instead of lemon

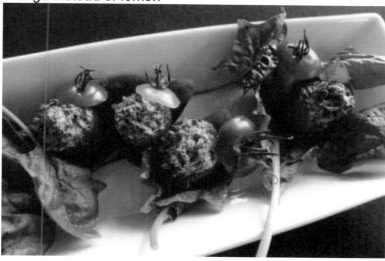

OYSTER MUSHROOMS

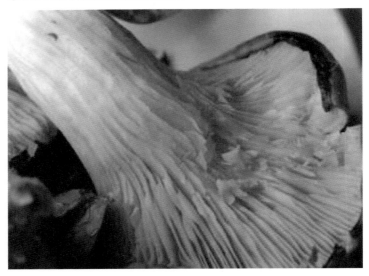

These beauties are grossly under-rated so I am here to sing their song! Who knew delicious could have so many health benefits!

-they reduce cholesterol via a compound they produce called statins, which signal the liver to clear out bad cholesterol, effectively lowering LDL

-they contain a specific polysaccharide called pleuron, which ongoing studies are finding to have an anti-tumor effect

-they absorb mercury and other toxins as they go through your system - you definitely want this food floating through your body and collecting all the toxins to flush out

Oyster mushrooms have their own distinct wonderful scent and mix well with all vegetables. Beetles do like them too though so be sure to carefully dry wipe them down completely before eating. *To your health*

STUFFED OLIVES & OYSTER MUSHROOMS

I always seem to be having long leisurely dinners, even when I am alone, with multiple courses; starters like this are always divine. They are full of flavor, extremely pleasing to the eye, wonderful for preparing the appetite for the courses to follow, and so light that they will never spoil the remainder of the meal. Also, the flavors are mild, with spices purposely omitted, truly making this the perfect complimentary opener.

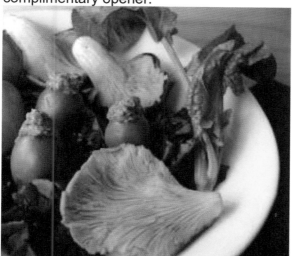

OLIVE STUFFING, IN FOOD PROCESSOR
1 cup spinach
½ cup fresh basil
2 tbsp ground flax
1 tsp nutritional yeast
1 clove garlic
½ cup pine nuts (or walnuts)
SERVE on a bed of spinach

VARIATION: by removing the ground flax and adding olive oil, you can easily create a salad dressing

RAINBOW SALAD

I can't talk health without talking rainbow salad. Nutrition is shockingly complex and shockingly simple at the same time. The fact is we can never understand the genius and complexity of food. We can keep studying and extracting bits & pieces of information, but we will never truly know everything there is to know - that's the complex part. The simple part is the fact that different fruits and vegetables all carry different components and by eating a large variety of these, we absorb more. Simple. Logical. We do know that different colors mean different nutrients so by incorporating as much color as possible you give your body more.

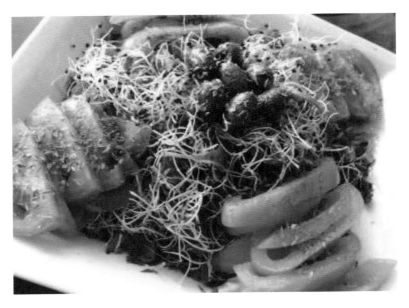

SALAD: chopped kale, collards, dill, purslane, parsley, rapini, spinach, mustard seed sprouts, vine ripened tomato, yellow bell pepper, Greek kalamata olives

DRESSING: Basil infused olive oil, paprika, pinch of cumin, juice of a lemon, and organic dried oregano.

RAINBOW EATING

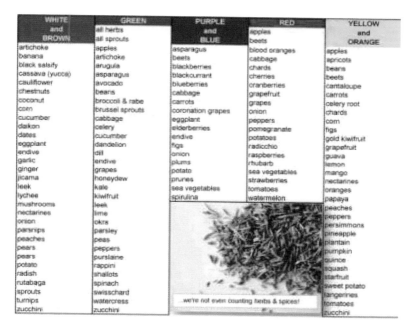

WHITE and BROWN	GREEN	PURPLE and BLUE	RED	YELLOW and ORANGE
artichoke	all herbs	asparagus	apples	apples
banana	all sprouts	beets	beets	apricots
black salsify	apples	blackberries	blood oranges	beans
cassava (yucca)	artichoke	blackcurrant	cabbage	beets
cauliflower	arugula	blueberries	chards	cantaloupe
chestnuts	asparagus	cabbage	cherries	carrots
coconut	avocado	carrots	cranberries	celery root
corn	beans	coronation grapes	grapefruit	chards
cucumber	broccoli & rabe	eggplant	grapes	corn
daikon	brussel sprouts	elderberries	onion	figs
dates	cabbage	endive	peppers	gold kiwifruit
eggplant	celery	figs	pomegranate	grapefruit
endive	cucumber	onion	potatoes	guava
garlic	dandelion	plums	radicchio	lemon
ginger	dill	potato	raspberries	mango
jicama	endive	prunes	rhubarb	nectarines
leek	grapes	sea vegetables	sea vegetables	oranges
lychee	honeydew	spirulina	strawberries	papaya
mushrooms	kale		tomatoes	peaches
nectarines	kiwifruit		watermelon	peppers
onion	leek			persimmons
parsnips	lime			pineapple
peaches	okra			plantain
pears	parsley			pumpkin
pears	peas			quince
potato	peppers			squash
radish	purslaine			starfruit
rutabaga	rappini			sweet potato
sprouts	shallots			tangerines
turnips	spinach			tomatoes
zucchini	swisschard			zucchini
	watercress			
	zucchini			

...we're not even counting herbs & spices!

You do not need to memorize this list – you never want to take the fun out of healthy eating. Instead, look at is as an exploration, a whole new world of recipes to discover! Make a game out of it...once a week pick something from this list you normally do not eat and then find a recipe that looks interesting. This would also work in the reverse. Let the colors of nature inspire you when you shop. Whatever exotic vegetable or fruit looks interesting to you, buy it! Then just do a search with that food + "recipe". You will be amazed at how many options come up! ...all of that variation is what you want. You don't even need to know exact nutrients, you just want to vary as many colors as often as possible and you'll be getting everything nature offers.

FEAST FOR THE EYES STARTER

Of course we all know greens are great for us, but they are not appealing to most people. I have yet to meet anyone who didn't love this starter…

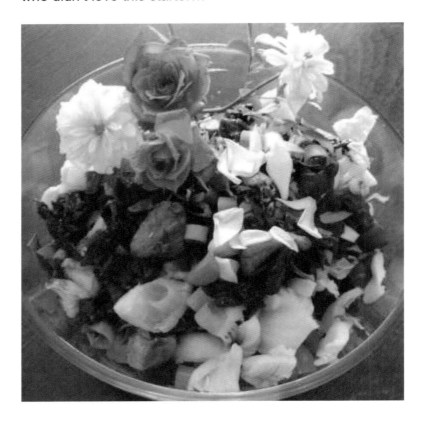

SALAD: watercress, baby greens, red swisschard, tat soi, fresh basil, arugula, spinach, red cabbage, sun dried tomatoes, oyster mushrooms, king mushrooms, green onion, edible flowers. Dressing is usually unnecessary given all the flavors – a sprinkle of sea salt, freshly cracked pepper, and juice of lemon or lime work really well

...it's all in the presentation...

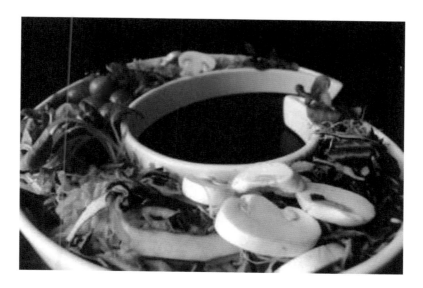

FLAVORFUL MEDITERRANEAN DRESSING

Juice of 2 limes
2 cloves raw garlic or 4 cloves roasted garlic
1 tbsp cumin powder
1 tsp cayenne pepper
1 tbsp fresh or dried oregano
1 tsp balsamic vinegar (adjust if you have aged)
8 tbsp olive oil
1/3 cup chopped sun dried tomatoes
1/4 cup chopped olives (black or green)
1 stalk chopped green onion
--Keeps in the refrigerator for 2-4 days

Between this awesome dressing and beautiful plating, you can get anyone to eat more greens!

MUSHROOM INSPIRED TAPAS

TAPAS is a word from Spain meaning many varied appetizers (cold & warm) and has gained popularity with "Tapas Bars" opening all over the world. It is a terrific way to get a taste of many different foods and enjoy the contrast of flavors. Even using the same topping, it will taste quite different if it is eaten with cool refreshing cucumber or hot red peppers.

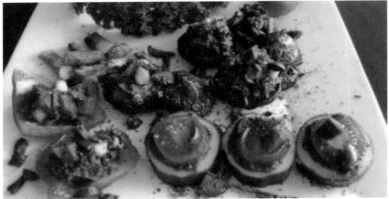

FOOD PROCESSOR OR HAND CHOPPED:

2 cups kale

1 cup parsley

1/4 cup tahini

1/4 cup black pitted olives

1/2 cup pre-soaked chia seeds (quinoa also great)

1/2 cup baby onion sprouts

2 cloves garlic

½ tsp chili pepper

juice of 1 lime + rinds

2 tbsp flax seed oil

1 tbsp nutritional yeast

top with chopped olives, shallot, dried or fresh oregano

--SERVE on mushrooms or any vegetables

DANDELION MIX ON PORTOBELLO MUSHROOM

While we're talking mushrooms... what a starter!

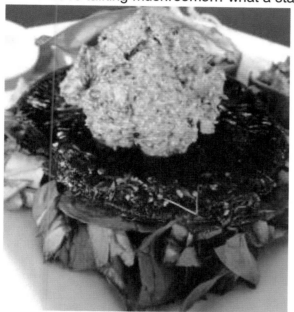

THE SPREAD: in a food processor combine 1 cup dandelion, 1 cup spinach, 1 cup brussel sprouts, 1 cup cilantro, ½ cup tahini, ¼ cup black pitted olives, juice of one orange (and 1 tsp rinds), 1 cup baby onion sprouts, 3 cloves garlic, ½ cup sea vegetables (I used arame here, can be any variety), 1 tbsp cayenne pepper, 4 tbsp flax seed oil, 2 tbsp nutritional yeast, 1 tbsp dried oregano
TIP: add a little water and it becomes a dip

THE PORTOBELLO: on very low heat (about 100 degrees) using coconut oil, sprinkle with cracked black pepper, a little Himalayan salt, and dried oregano or thyme – just for a moment on each side.

COLLARDS, PURE LIFE

Collards are pure life, pure power, pure nutrition.
(per 100g)
Vitamin A: 575mg (64% of RDA)
Vitamin C: 26mg (43%)
Vitamin K: 623mcg (593%)
Calcium: 210mg (21%)
Collards are eaten all over the world and are a green that have so many different names throughout so many different cultures. We may call it by different names, but its power is undisputed.

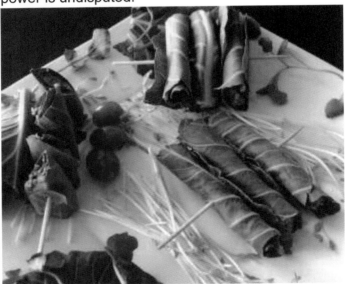

Not only a nutrient powerhouse and beautiful to look at, collards have the perfect sturdy texture for wraps. Roll them extra small to turn them into cocktail bites.

Shown here with the dandelion mixture from the previous page, when served as cocktail food, even the most hesitant vegetable eater won't be able to resist.

GREAT LITTLE TRICK TO GET MORE GREENS

Collard greens are powerful all on their own, but if you want to add even more to that, here's a terrific little trick that also makes your wrap even more sturdy and easier to transport if you are packing a lunch: line it up with spinach leaves before putting everything else in. And if you are transporting, remember to fold the ends in before you roll.

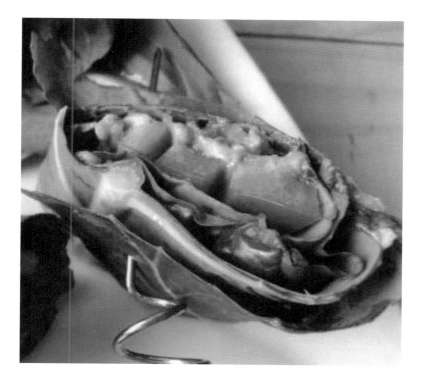

This is another terrific opportunity to add sprouts as well.

Layering in nutrition to wraps, sandwiches, lasagna, tomato towers,... is really easy – it's just a question of remembering to do it.

MAKI – there are no rules

I've never been good at following rules in life and I see no reason why it would be different with food. One of the best things you can do in your kitchen is forget everything you were ever taught and create on your own.

The fact is "maki" in Japanese means rolling. *...no one ever specified rolling what...* It's fun to get ideas and inspiration from recipes, but when it comes to making food on a daily basis – roam free and let your mind wander, use whatever flavors you really love, whatever appeals to you.

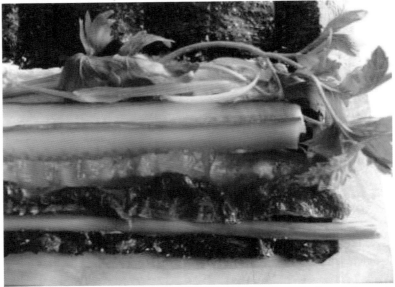

DECONSTRUCTED: Spread hummus on nori sheet (good old fashioned chick pea hummus that usually leaves leftovers to do exactly this with)
-Cucumber, green onion, sun dried tomatoes, green tomatoes (less watery than red and will hold up better in a roll), parsley (I have used every green known to man)

YELLOW ZUCCHINI AND CILANTRO ROLLS

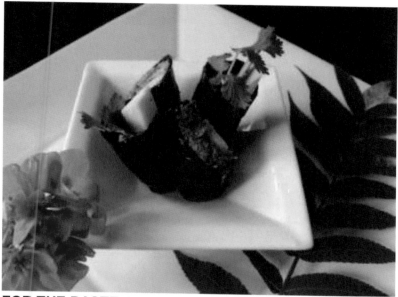

FOR THE PASTE, IN FOOD PROCESSOR:

2 cups arugula

1 cup cilantro

1/2 cup walnuts

2 cloves garlic

1 small onion

3 oz sun dried tomato

1/2 cup tahini

Juice of 1 lime

2 tbsp ground flax seeds

1 tbsp nutritional yeast

1 tsp cayenne

IN ROLL: use strips of yellow zucchini and cilantro

...as you can see, anything goes. Wrap tight and small, cut into bite sized smaller pieces and it's appetizer heaven!

CHOP SALADS

One of the bad habits many people have is how they define "appetizer" or "starter". It is usually something battered and fried and starts you off on the wrong foot right at the beginning of the meal.

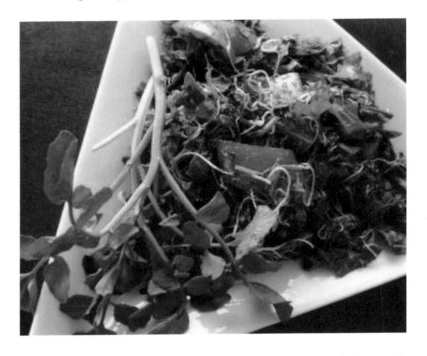

Start looking at a chop salad like this one as a starter and you will instantly boost your health right up!

RECIPE: Chopped watercress, arugula, purslane, red peppers, sprouts, sea vegetables (dulse), garlic, cayenne pepper, flaxseed oil, freshly squeezed juice of an orange (instead of lemon/lime, this will add sweetness and balance the slightly bitter taste of the watercress as well as work with the cayenne in covering the sea vegetable taste)

I love chop salads – besides the fact that they are easier to eat than when the greens are large pieces, they create versatility. A finely chopped salad easily becomes a salsa and ready for dipping, or it can be a stuffing for peppers or mushrooms, it can act as a topping, and so on. Versatility is a really great thing in the kitchen because it lets you take something and modify it as needed or just gives your overall menu more variety.

The other reason I love chop salads is that they make it easy to hide flavors. Not everyone likes the taste of say, sea vegetables, or certain other foods... dandelion can be bitter... but we know they're good for us... by adding them into a salad that has a mix of many other flavors + strong spices, the "disliked" flavor goes completely unnoticed.

Handy little trick.

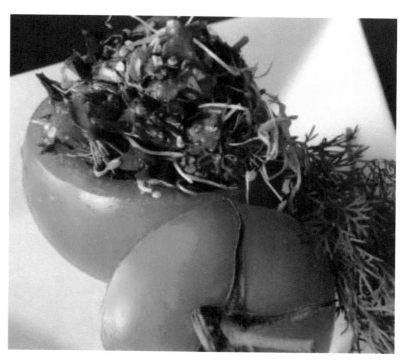

Copyright © 2012 Black Wave Publishing

All rights reserved. Reproduction in any manner without written permission is prohibited except for brief quotations for review or media purposes.

Library and Archives Canada

Author: Karr, Jaqui

Title: Fast, Simple & Fresh Gluten Free Recipes for Soups & Appetizers Deliciously Engineered for Weight Loss

ISBN: 978-0-9869039-6-0

Publication Date: April 13, 2012

This book should not be used for diagnosing or treating medical issues. Always consult a trained medical professional with regards to health problems.

2474976R00026

Printed in Germany
by Amazon Distribution
GmbH, Leipzig